MoonTime Magic

How to Transform Your Period into Your Favorite Time of the Month

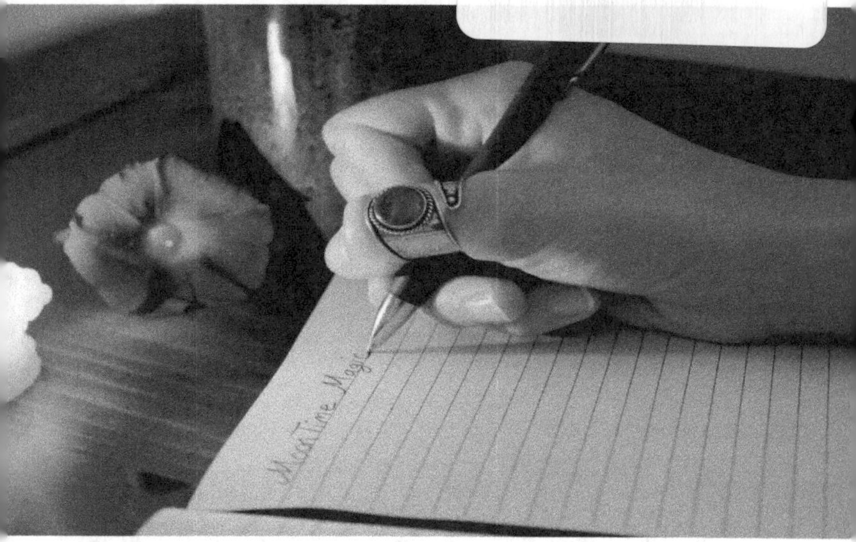

By Briar Accalia

ISBN-13: 978-1537735931
ISBN-10: 1537735934

To Sven and Riley.
Always.

Table of Contents

"The great mother whom we call Innana gave a gift to woman that is not known among men, and this is the secret of blood. The flow at the dark of the moon, the healing blood of the moon's birth- to men, this is flux and distemper, bother and pain. They imagine we suffer and consider themselves lucky. We do not disabuse them.

In the red tent, the truth is known. In the red tent, where days pass like a gentle stream, as the gift of Innana courses through us, cleansing the body of last month's death, preparing the body to receive the new month's life, women give thanks — for repose and restoration, for the knowledge that life comes from between our legs, and that life costs blood."

—Anita Diamant, *The Red Tent*

Chapter 1:

Culture and The Menstrual Cycle

What comes to mind when you think of your first-ever menstrual period (menarche)? What was your experience like? If you're like most women, there was probably a lot of secrecy, embarrassment, or shame around it. Your mother may have expressed sympathy that you would now have to deal with this "nasty" inconvenience every single month for the next 30ish years. You may have been ostracized by your male friends and ignored by your father. You may have felt horrified that you were now officially growing up.

I started my period at school when I was eleven years old. I realized it quickly and stuffed some toilet paper into my underwear to soak up the blood and went about the rest of my day like nothing had happened. I was embarrassed- so much so that I didn't even tell my mom for the first few days, but instead went into her bathroom when she wasn't home and took some of her pads to use. When I finally worked up the courage to tell her, she acknowledged it uncomfortably and bought me my own pads. I assume she may have told my dad that I had started my period, but he never said anything about it. That was about the extent of it. It was a bit devastating for me to become a woman, especially being a "tomboy" who spent most of my childhood wishing I was a boy.

In our culture, this kind of neutral or negative reaction to the menstrual cycle is the norm. We're taught to be embarrassed about our bleeding each month, so we try our hardest to hide it, lie about it, pretend it just doesn't exist. This is really obvious in the marketing for "feminine hygiene products." Just that name is euphemistic and implies that the bleeding is inherently dirty and disgusting. The focus is on small tampons that you can hide discreetly in your pocket so that no one will know what you're going into the bathroom to do. There's a focus on tampons and pads that are so "effective" that you can continue your normal, high-energy activities, even participate in intense sports without having to be interrupted by something like your uterus bleeding for days.

This attitude is unfortunate, because in reality, our cycles, and our bleeding in particular, are powerful tools if we know how to use them. This is where our creativity comes from, our ability to birth- not just birth babies, but any kind of idea, project, or creation. It's an opportunity to connect to nature since our cycles follow the moon, and it's an opportunity to connect to our truest selves and to our intuition. Going along with the culture in hiding it, viewing it as gross, being embarrassed about it and teaching our daughters to be embarrassed about it, is perpetuating an outdated system that's no longer needed. It's perpetuating a fear and suppression of women's power and autonomy that's left over from the days of the witch trials. Let's finally heal from that and move on.

Many women have troubles with their menstrual cycle because of physical issues- things like cramps and PMS.

These are legitimate issues that can usually be remedied naturally with a little bit of patience and an open mind. Lifestyle is extremely important when it comes to having a good menstrual cycle, and it involves more than just diet and exercise. It's not difficult, though- it's actually more enjoyable than how you're probably living now! You can lower your stress, be more efficient in your work, improve your relationships, and decrease cramps and mood swings. This is what I'll be teaching you in this book!

I mentioned before that the female cycle follows the moon. Let me explain what I mean by this and offer something very practical that you can do to start improving your cycle.

No one really knows why, but women used to bleed with the new moon and ovulate with the full moon. Female cycles were (and still mostly are) the same length as one orbit of the moon around the Earth- about 29 days. Nature reuses things that work, so you find recurring patterns everywhere. My guess is that there's some evolutionary pattern that's been handed down since before we were mammals and still lived in water, where we would be strongly affected by the tides. Something about reproduction cycles in those creatures have simply remained in the same pattern since that time.

Once we started disconnecting from nature, and especially after artificial light was invented and widely used, that pattern started being disrupted. Artificial light causes our hormones to become imbalanced, which can have some drastic effects on our menstrual cycles. Since light at inappropriate times causes our hormones to be imbalanced, lining up your cycle with the moon can do more than just that: it can also help with things like irregular menstrual cycles, PMS, PCOS, and infertility since those problems are also caused by hormone imbalances. If you want to line up your cycle with the moon, follow these simple steps:

1. Make your bedroom completely dark. This means using black-out shades, or perhaps black trash bags or something of the sort, over your windows. Put a towel under the door to block out light. Make sure you don't have a lit clock or any electronics with blinking lights. Really try to make it absolutely black. If you need to use the bathroom in the middle of the night and need a light, get a red night light.

2. For just three days of the month- the day before the full moon, the day of the full moon, and the day after the full moon- sleep with a light on. A dim lamp will do, or a hall or

closet light with the door cracked. This mimics the light of the full moon.

After a few months, you may notice that your cycle is nearly lined up: you'll be ovulating with the full moon and bleeding with the new moon. You'll need to do this consistently to continue having balanced hormones and aligning with the moon. A simple alternative would be to sleep outside without lights, weather and location permitting!

Chapter 2:

Female Biology Crash Course

Most people don't really learn about what's physically happening throughout the monthly female cycle because there's such a taboo around it. That's slowly changing, and if you're reading this book right now, you're on the front edge of it by being brave enough and open enough to start overcoming your conditioning towards it and embracing it as a natural, normal, and powerful part of being a female. I'm not a biologist so I'll only go over the basics of this and the practical aspects. This isn't going to be an extensive, complicated science lesson, it's just to give you a working knowledge of what's going on in the big picture so that you can better understand the rest of the book.

The Physiology

There are four phases to each monthly cycle. Since it's a cycle, it's a little difficult to just pick a point to start, but I think it will make the most sense when we're talking about the physiology to start in the follicular phase.

1. Follicular Phase

The follicular phase is the time between bleeding and ovulation. So you've stopped bleeding, but you haven't ovulated yet. Two hormones are rising: estrogen and follicle-stimulating hormone (FSH). FSH stimulates about twelve eggs to grow inside the follicles. A follicle is a kind of shell that the egg grows inside within the ovaries. Hence why it's called the follicular phase- the follicles and eggs are maturing. Once the eggs have matured some, they start releasing estrogen. Estrogen starts to build up the uterine lining, which is the layer of blood lining the uterus that gives a fertilized egg a place to implant into if you get pregnant.

2. Ovulatory Phase

Next is the ovulatory phase. During this phase, a hormone called luteinizing hormone (LH) spikes and then drops just as quickly, and this is what actually releases the egg from the follicle and the ovary. Estrogen also peaks here and testosterone increases, so your sex drive goes up and there are subtle or not-so-subtle changes in your appearance and behavior. Just a few fun facts: when women are in their ovulatory phase, they tend to shop more, spending more money on beauty products, clothes, jewelry, and such. Also, they tend to avoid their fathers more, even to the point of talking to them less on the phone, which is probably an instinctual way to avoid incest.

3. Luteal Phase

Third is the luteal phase, which is after you've ovulated and before you start bleeding. Estrogen stays high at first but then starts to drop, and the empty follicle starts producing a hormone called progesterone, which takes over for the rest of the cycle. Progesterone stabilizes that lining in the uterus and makes it more like a sponge for a fertilized egg to potentially implant into.

4. Menstrual Phase

Last is the menstrual phase, which is when you're bleeding. If an egg has not been fertilized, estrogen and progesterone both drop really quickly, which causes the lining of blood in the uterus to be shed as your period. If an egg has been fertilized, it will nest into that lining and you'll continue producing progesterone so that the lining will stay and the baby can grow, and you will no longer have a menstrual cycle going on.

A more practical detail is the tool that you use during your period to hold your blood. Most women wear normal tampons, but you may want to rethink that. Conventional tampons and pads have a massive amount of chemicals in them, from pesticides used on the cotton to plasticizing chemicals to chemical fragrances. These chemicals are all put in or on your vagina, which is a highly sensitive area. It's extremely absorbent, and these chemicals are basically going directly into your bloodstream. Some of them are endocrine disruptors, meaning they mess with your hormones.

Fortunately, there are alternatives. Many health food stores, including Whole Foods, have organic or chemical-free versions of disposable tampons and pads. They're more expensive, but they're totally worth it if you prefer having something that you can just throw away when you're done with it.

Another option that's less expensive in the long run and a lot more "earthy" is to get organic cotton or hemp cloth pads. I really like these because I get to be more intimately involved in my cycle through washing them at the end of my bleeding time. It's like a ritual for me. I don't like wearing tampons because it feels like I'm just plugging up my cycle and pretending it's not there, so it's harder for me to get in touch with the power of bleeding and my intuition. One more option is menstrual cups. A menstrual cup is literally a little cup, usually silicone, that you put into the vagina that holds the blood until it's full. The cool thing about these is that you can then do things with the blood- if you have houseplants or a garden, the blood is a really good fertilizer. I haven't personally used a menstrual cup yet, but women who do use them seem to really like them. You can also use the soaking water from cloth pads to water plants.

Tracking

Now that you know what's happening during each phase, let's ground it into your own personal reality by learning how you can recognize and track where you're at in your cycle.

If you have a regular cycle of about 29 days, then you can estimate generally when these four phases will be. It's easiest to start with the menstrual phase, since that's a very obvious sign of when a phase is starting. The first day of bleeding marks the first day of your menstrual phase. This phase will last as long as you're bleeding, usually about 3-7 days. After that is the follicular phase, which lasts from the end of bleeding until about day 14. Day 14 is about when you ovulate. Ovulation is technically more of an event than an extended phase, so it's really only a day, occasionally two days. When you're scheduling things to do during each phase (more on that in the next chapter), you can extend the ovulatory phase out to a few more days, even a week, because your estrogen will still be high, so your mood and strengths will be very similar. Then, the luteal phase is simply from after ovulation until you start bleeding again.

If you want to know more precisely when your phases are, you'll have to figure out exactly when you ovulate. The method that I'll be teaching here is part of something called fertility awareness. Full fertility awareness is normally used for birth control or family planning purposes, but I won't be going into the details of that- I'll just be telling you how to use the basics of it to track where you're at in your cycle. Even though I use it to avoid conception and I would definitely recommend it if you think it's right for you, I am by no means an expert in this area, so if you want to start actually using this as a way to avoid pregnancy, please do your own detailed research, get good at it before ditching other methods of birth control, and perhaps visit someone who's trained in it so they can help you learn the nuances of your own unique cycle. If you'd rather use other methods of birth control, that's perfectly fine- you can still use fertility awareness alongside it just to gain a better understanding of your body.

Again, it's generally pretty obvious when your period starts and stops, so you've got the menstrual and follicular phases covered. To figure out ovulation, you'll need to keep track of at least one of two things: your basal body temperature and your cervical mucus.

Basal Body Temperature

Basal body temperature is simply your temperature before you get out of bed in the morning. Keep a thermometer right next to your bed every night and take your temperature before you even stand up. It's best if you wake up at the same time every day, because your temperature will fluctuate depending on the time. It will also fluctuate if you've had a bad night's sleep, if you're sick, or if you were drinking alcohol the night before. When you're charting your temperatures, you'll see that before ovulation, your temperature is a little lower, maybe in the mid to upper 97s or lower 98s. As a side note, if it's consistently lower than mid 97s, it's possible that you might have an issue with hypothyroidism, so if that's a pattern that you see, you might want to look into it to see if you have any of the symptoms and get tested.

After ovulation, progesterone causes your temperature to go up and stay up for the rest of the cycle. This is because your body is trying to create a very warm environment for a possible baby. It should go up by at least 2/10ths of a degree higher than it has been the previous six days. If it looks like your temperature jumps up, look back at your previous week's temperatures and find the highest one. Today's temperature should be 2/10ths of a degree or more higher than that one, and it should remain that way for at least three days. The day that you actually ovulated was probably the day before your temperature jumped up. If it goes up for a few days and then starts dropping again, you may have a problem with low progesterone. If your temperature didn't go up and stay up at all your whole cycle and it can't be explained by inconsistent waking times or illness, then you didn't ovulate. Lack of ovulation is a sign of hormone imbalance (unless you're breastfeeding or approaching menopause) and is a message that you need to improve your lifestyle. Aligning your cycle with the moon as described in the last chapter and following the rest of the advice in the book should help any kind of hormone imbalance you may have.

Cervical Mucus

The other way to find out when you ovulate is to keep track of your cervical mucus. This is harder to do just because it's more interpretive than taking your temperature, but basically, before ovulation you'll be drier and any cervical mucus you have will feel sticky or creamy, like glue or lotion. Then, when you ovulate, the mucus will be slippery and like egg whites, so if you take some between two fingers and then slowly pull your fingers apart, the mucus will stretch between your fingers. When you have stretchy mucus like this and then for the next few days it's sticky or creamy or dry, then you'll know that you ovulated on that stretchy mucus day.

If you have more questions about fertility awareness or want to know more about using it to either prevent pregnancy or to know when to get pregnant, then I highly recommend the book Honoring Our Cycles by Katie Singer. There are also practitioners who are experienced in knowing what all the weird things mean, the things that might not quite fit the descriptions that I've just given, because everybody is different. You might have mucus that doesn't fit the most common descriptions, and that can still be normal for you. But as long as you're ovulating, then this should work to let you know when it's happening and get more connected to your body.

"..by honouring the demands of our bleeding, our blood gives us something in return. The crazed bitch from irritation hell recedes. In her place arises a side of ourselves with whom we may not-at first- be comfortable. She is a vulnerable, highly perceptive genius who can ponder a given issue and take her world by storm. When we're quiet and bleeding, we stumble upon solutions to dilemmas that've been bugging us all month. Inspiration hits and moments of epiphany rumba 'cross de tundra of our senses. In this mode of existence one does not feel antipathy towards a bodily ritual that so profoundly and routinely reinforces our cuntpower. "

—Inga Muscio, *Cunt: A Declaration of Independence*

Chapter 3:

Planning Your Month

To recap the phases: there's the menstrual phase, when you're bleeding; the follicular phase, between bleeding and ovulation; the ovulatory phase, when you're ovulating; and the luteal phase, which is between ovulation and bleeding, and is otherwise known as PMS week or hell week. Or two weeks.

I'll now go into a little more depth with these four phases and talk about our strengths during each phase. By scheduling our month so that we do certain things during each phase- things that we'll naturally be best at during that phase- we'll be much happier and more effective. We can improve our stress levels, our work lives, and our relationships. I'll go through each phase one by one and show you how you can work with your body to make every month a more pleasurable and productive experience.

The Menstrual Phase

First, the menstrual phase. While most women in our culture dread starting their period every month, this is actually my favorite time of the month because of the way I take care of myself and the way I can connect with myself.

The menstrual phase is when the two hemispheres of your brain are able to best communicate, so this is a great time to listen to your intuition and make connections where you may not have seen them before. It's a time to reflect on yourself and your life and figure out what your deepest desires are and then set intentions based on those desires. It's a time to be more introverted, not a time to be going to parties or serving others beyond what's necessary as far as children and whatnot. Make sure to make it a practice to have alone time where you can just sit and reflect. Do things that feel good and comforting- maybe journaling, reading a good book, drinking hot tea, painting or creative crafts. Don't feel like you always have to be doing anything, because you don't have much energy during the menstrual phase. Accept as much help as possible and allow others to nurture you. If you have a really amazing partner, ask him to do the cooking and housework for you this week (if you manage to do that, please let me know how). If it's possible, schedule your work life so that you're not as busy at this time of the month. It's not the time to finally get started on the 20-page report that's due at work tomorrow; you should have done it two weeks ago in your ovulatory phase. Of course, if the place you work isn't as flexible and you don't have a month to do a project, you may just have to do some things in a less-than-ideal phase, but wherever possible, schedule your month so that this time isn't as busy.

Some extra practices for the menstrual phase:

I really like oracle cards, and I have a goddess oracle card deck. Menstruation is a time to connect to your spirituality, whether you view that as god, goddess, intuition, universe, spirit, or whatever. Oracle cards help me recognize the goddess archetypes within me and draw forward each one's power as I need it. It helps me set intentions, things to focus on for the coming month. You could also use tarot cards or whatever you're comfortable using.

Another practice I like is journaling, and you can do this however you want. Just write what's on your mind, write what's on your heart, without censoring it, and you just might make connections you wouldn't have made otherwise. It can also be helpful to keep another journal throughout your whole cycle where you keep track of things like the food you're eating, your mood, any symptoms you're having, your activity level, and where in your cycle you're at. I've made downloads for journals like this that are available in my online course.

The Follicular Phase

Second is the follicular phase. This is the transition between bleeding and ovulation, from low to high energy, from internal to external, so this is when you're starting to feel more social, more juicy, more optimistic, more alive. This is when you'll enjoy going out with friends and going to concerts or other higher-energy events. It's the perfect time for creative problem solving, so if there's an issue that needs to be solved at work or in your relationship, it'll be easy to find solutions during this phase. The follicular phase is the time to actually plan for those desires that you tapped into during your bleeding time. You also might be more open to nurturing other people during this phase, and your sexuality will be increasing.

The Ovulatory Phase

Third is the ovulatory phase, when an egg is released from your ovaries. You'll be at the height of your energy and your sexuality in this phase, and you'll also have the best verbal skills out of the whole month. This means that the ovulatory phase is the best time to have important conversations, write important things, go on dates, continue being social and going out with friends. You'll probably want to actually get shit done during this phase. You'll be at the top of your game at work, both in your efficiency and in your popularity with coworkers. Personally, I've noticed that I love babies during this time and am quite nurturing, which of course makes sense because it's when I would actually be able to conceive.

The Luteal Phase

Last is the luteal phase, the week before your period where PMS kicks in for so many women. You're transitioning the other way now, from high to low energy, from external to internal, from nurturing others to nurturing yourself. If you have anger, irritability, sensitivity, etc., they're there for a reason. You're hypersensitive right now to actual injustices or things that aren't working for you in your life. It's time to notice those things. Write them down so that you'll remember them, notice patterns, and deal with them at the appropriate time in your cycle. This in itself will help to decrease the PMS because it's starting a cascade: as long as you notice the issues or the problems in your life during this phase, then reflect on them in the menstrual phase, find solutions for them in the follicular phase, and then act on them in the ovulatory phase, you'll be clearing out a lot of these issues that are in your subconscious the rest of the month, so there won't be as much to get "bitchy" about. You'll be implementing the solutions to all the recurring things you're getting upset about in this phase every month. Those issues will be gone because you're not just pushing them out of your mind during the rest of the month; instead, you're taking advantage of your strengths during each phase to make your life better.

When the emotions do come up in the luteal phase, which they inevitably will, since you're not really in a place to solve them right then and there, you don't just want to stuff them away. Instead, you can help release them in the moment by releasing through your body. Do something physical, such as: scream into a pillow or in your car, punch your bed, or dance without thinking about how you're dancing- just let your body do what it wants to do. Maybe it would feel good to do some yoga. Whatever feels right for that particular emotion is what you should do, as long as you use your body to release it and it doesn't harm you or anyone else.

The luteal phase is a time to start slowing down again. Be by yourself more, take good care of yourself by eating well, take baths or other things that feel nurturing and that you enjoy. Start accepting more help from others. The first half of this phase is a good time to take care of any mundane chores or errands.

Chapter 4:
Eating For Your Cycle

To have a healthy cycle, you have to be eating healthily. The food you consume literally becomes what your cells are made of, and it becomes the building blocks of your hormones, which of course control your cycle. I could write a whole book about nutrition, but in this one I'll just give some basics that are directly relevant to the menstrual cycle.

There are some things you should do throughout the month that will help you have a more balanced cycle. One of the major ones is to cut out processed foods: the sugar, white flour, soy, and vegetable oils and everything that's made with them- cookies, crackers, pizza, donuts, most breads, pasta, etc. If you want things like cookies and bread, my advice is to make them at home with properly prepared whole grains (more on that soon) or grain alternatives like amaranth, almond flour, and coconut flour (NOT potato or tapioca starch or flours made from legumes). Replace all the processed foods with foods you minimally process yourself at home, using ingredients that are whole, natural, fresh foods.

Avoid sugar like the plague, especially if you suffer from PMS. Women who suffer from PMS consume a whopping 275% more sugar than women who don't suffer from PMS. Correlation doesn't necessarily imply causation, but in this case, it makes sense because of what we know about the effects of sugar: sugar increases inflammation, which will make cramps worse; it sends your blood sugar on a roller coaster ride, which can cause irritability and mood swings; and it increases cortisol, the stress hormone, which then has downstream effects on the sex hormones and therefore the regularity and health of your cycle. It's really imperative to avoid refined sugar as much as you can. Moderate amounts of fruit and natural sweeteners like honey and maple syrup might be ok for you, it's just something you'll have to experiment with yourself and see if it works for you.

A couple other things that you might want to experiment with if you have PMS or cramps is to temporarily stop eating gluten and/or dairy. A lot of women don't do well with dairy because it can cause things like cramps, bloating and acne. With some people, it's only pasteurized dairy that causes a problem, and things like raw milk or raw cheeses don't bother them. These are much better for you anyway. Pasteurization has problems beyond just the menstrual cycle. My suggestion is to cut out all dairy for at least a full cycle, which is hard, but you can get through it. Notice if your cramps were any less severe than usual or if you were less irritable than usual, or anything out of the ordinary. Then, reintroduce some raw dairy- eat it alone- and see if any symptoms come up. If they do, you know dairy is a problem for you and it's something you should avoid.

Concerning gluten, I personally don't think gluten in and of itself is actually a problem for most people (though of course there are people who have an actual allergy or intolerance to any amount of gluten itself). I say that because many of the people who don't do well with modern wheat do perfectly well with ancient varieties of wheat, such as einkorn, that are properly prepared by soaking or sour-leavening, like in sourdough bread. Grains, nuts, seeds and beans should all be soaked before cooking them in order to inactivate something called phytic acid, which binds to minerals in the digestive tract and makes you deficient in those minerals. If you want to know more about exactly how to do that, there's tons of information about it online, and there's an awesome cookbook called Nourishing Traditions by Sally Fallon of the Weston A Price Foundation. Gluten is just another thing you'll have to experiment with. I suggest doing the same procedure that I outlined for experimenting with dairy- cut it out for a full cycle and see how you feel, then reintroduce an ancient variety of wheat that you've soaked and see how you feel.

So now that you know what you might need to avoid, what should you eat in order to start having a healthy menstrual cycle? Here are some of the most important nutrients for your menstrual cycle and what foods are highest in those nutrients:

-Vitamin A: grass-fed butter, egg yolks, liver, seafood, cod liver oil

-Vitamin B6: raw animal products, liver, starchy veggies, fruit, blackstrap molasses

-Vitamin B12: animal products esp. red meat

-Vitamin D: sunlight, butter, eggs, liver, seafood (shrimp), cod liver oil

-Calcium: dairy, bone broth, fish with bones, dark leafy greens, sesame seeds, blackstrap molasses

-Magnesium: broth, cacao, most other foods (whole grains, leafy greens, nuts and seeds)

-Zinc: oysters, red meat, nuts, seeds, beans, ginger

-Omega 3s:

   -DHA: fatty fish (salmon, anchovies, mackerel), grass-fed meat, liver, algae

   -GLA: evening primrose, borage, and black currant oils; hemp seeds, oats, barley, spirulina

   You want to be eating these and other nutrients all month long, but they're especially important in the luteal phase, because you have increased nutrient requirements at that time. As a side note, please don't be afraid of animal products or saturated fat. All the "science" against that is essentially junk science funded by the major food companies. All they care about is making money, they do not care about your health. A good book about this that goes over all the history and science of the low-fat agenda is called Big Fat Suprise by Nina Teicholz. Saturated fat is actually necessary for building and balancing hormones, among other things, and as I've stated before, building and balancing hormones is essential for a healthy cycle.

For the menstrual phase in particular, you'll want to continue eating the foods I just mentioned, and also make sure to focus on the following two nutrients:

-Iron: red meat, liver, clams, leafy greens
-Vitamin C: colorful plant foods, especially wild foods (garlic mustard, lamb's quarters, white pine needle tea, etc.), red bell peppers, citrus, leafy greens

Getting enough bioavailable iron is important since you're losing blood, and vitamin C helps you absorb iron (calcium inhibits the absorption of iron, so try to eat high-iron and high-calcium foods at different meals). Wild foods are really easy to find in your backyard, and they're free! Just make sure to positively identify any wild edible, of course. Use more than one field guide plus online sources.

During your follicular and ovulatory phases, your specific nutrient requirements aren't quite as high, but it's still important to eat well of course. It's ok here to eat a little bit lighter, maybe not quite as much red meat, and a little more dairy if that agrees with you. And of course, continue avoiding sugar and processed foods.

I strongly suggest that you find the best sourcing for your food as possible. Go to your local farmers market where you'll be able to talk to the farmer and ask questions. The food will be so much fresher, and most of them won't be spraying their plants with chemicals or injecting their animals with antibiotics and hormones. The animals should be outside for as much of the year as possible and eating a biologically appropriate diet. Cows should be eating grass and hay, not corn and chicken feces. Chickens and pigs are both omnivores so it's okay for them to eat supplemental grain, but they should also be pecking or rooting around outside for vegetation and bugs. It's fine if your local farmer isn't certified organic- most small farmers can't afford the certification process, but their food will be higher quality than the certified organic food that's coming out of huge monoculture operations in California.

I don't generally recommend supplements. Your body doesn't recognize synthetic nutrients very well, so all you'll end up with is expensive urine (since you'll be excreting most of it). If you know that you're very deficient in a lot of nutrients, supplements made from whole foods can be helpful temporarily to give you a boost, but you should always be aiming to improve your diet to the point that you're getting everything you need from just food. It's often said that in our modern world we can't get everything we need from just food, but that's only true if you're eating poor quality food. If you follow the sourcing that I just went over, you'll be good- this type of ecologically raised food is far superior nutritionally to anything you'll find in the supermarket. If for some reason you absolutely cannot or will not source most of your food well, or if you've been eating nothing but a standard American diet all your life, then a multivitamin made from whole foods is totally understandable.

The one supplement that I do recommend is fermented cod liver oil. It's really high in vitamins A and D, plus it has some omega 3 fats and vitamin K. Most people are quite deficient in these nutrients, and cod liver oil is a very natural, traditional source of them.

Overall, make sure you're getting a variety of whole foods throughout the month, ideally including organs and seafood, red meat, lots of colorful vegetables and greens, supplemented with some properly prepared whole grains, nuts, seeds, and dairy- preferably raw- if it agrees with you. Focus on the richer animal foods and the greens and other colorful veggies during your luteal and menstrual phases. Experiment to see what feels good and what doesn't. Keep a food journal so that you can start to see connections between what you eat and how it affects your cycle.

Chapter 5:

Moving Around Your Cycle

When it comes to your cycle and every other aspect of your life, movement is an essential thing to optimize. Exercise will raise levels of endorphins, which can get low during the luteal phase. It will also help clear out toxins and excess hormones from your body, and it lowers inflammation. Movement pretty much helps everything. We're designed as human beings on this planet to be active throughout the day. As women, evolutionarily speaking, our bodies have adapted to being outside foraging for a good portion of the day, which would involve a lot of walking, squatting down to dig up plants, and load bearing- carrying baskets, water, firewood, children and whatnot.

You don't have to be an elite athlete to be healthy. One thing that bothers me about modern research is that most of it is done on and geared towards men. These studies always say that the best kind of exercise is high-intensity interval training (HIIT) a couple times a week, where you alternate between a short period of really high intensity exercise and a period of recovery. So for example, you would sprint all-out for 30 seconds, then walk for 60 seconds, and you'd do that a few times. I'm not saying exercise like that is unhealthy for women, but there have been studies showing that for women, it's just as effective to do lower-intensity things like walking, gardening, etc. and to me, that makes sense from an evolutionary perspective. Intuitively, I feel like the most beneficial things for women will be walking, squatting, and carrying loads. If you have other goals besides general health and longevity, such as weight loss or muscle gain, or if you just enjoy more intense exercise, then yes, add in more intense exercise. It's probably good for all of us to do on occasion just for the sheer variety. Just do most of it in the right time of the month- the follicular and ovulatory phases. In the luteal and menstrual phases, you'll probably want to back off and go to the lower-intensity things, unless you're just really feeling it that day. Always listen to your body.

Another related thing with exercise that I'd like to spell out here in case it wasn't implied enough already is that you should aim to not just exercise for half an hour a day and then sit around on your ass the rest of the day. It'll be most helpful if you stay at a low level of activity for most of the day doing things like walking, gardening or housework. You can even just switch up positions while you're at work or doing whatever you do at home, like going from sitting to standing to kneeling. There are endless ways to sit, stand, and kneel- be creative! Park further away in the parking lot while running errands and take stairs instead of elevators. Always try to sneak in a little more movement throughout your day. Always try to get movement variety into your life just like you should be getting nutritional variety.

A lot of that variety can be spread out throughout your cycle. You should always have that baseline of daily movement, but then you can add things on or make adjustments based on where you're at in your cycle and how you're feeling.

During the menstrual phase, since you'll have lower energy, you'll want to take it easy, even on the baseline level. Still do some easy movement, like gentle yoga at home or slow walks outside. Make sure your body gets plenty of rest, though, that's what it's asking for. You'll probably want to do these things alone, otherwise you may get drained or irritated.

During the ovulatory phase, you can get as intense as you want. Don't overdo it to the point where it's painful or dangerous, but if you have the energy to lift weights, do high intensity interval training, go dancing or running, play a sport, or whatever else you're into, then go for it. You'll probably also enjoy exercising with other people during this phase, so if you can do that, all the better.

The follicular and luteal phases should be transitions between the other phases. During the follicular phase, you're starting to gain more energy, so you can start increasing the intensity during this phase. During the luteal phase, your energy is decreasing, so start decreasing the intensity as well.

Chapter 6:

PMS: How to Not Feel Like You're Dying

The dreaded "hell week." So many women struggle with PMS during the luteal phase, and it just doesn't have to be that way. There are a lot of doctors who dismiss PMS, saying it's just part of being a woman, and prescribe birth control pills or antidepressants with dangerous side effects. These don't address the root cause of the issue- they just cover up symptoms IF they even work at all. Fortunately, you don't have to live with PMS.

Just to be clear, I'm not saying that during your luteal phase you'll feel exactly the same as you feel in your ovulatory phase, because you won't. It IS normal in your luteal phase for your energy to start dropping and for you to start being sensitive to the things that aren't serving you. It's NOT normal for you to feel completely bat-shit crazy every month, where one second you're having an orgasm over a piece of chocolate, the next second you're crying over a dog food commercial, and the next second you're chasing your partner around the house with a knife. That was possibly a little exaggerated, but I'm sure we can all relate.

There's basically one issue at work when it comes to PMS: not listening to your body-mind's signals. Your body-mind's signals include the increased emotional sensitivity, the mood swings, and the physical symptoms like cramps- all the things that happen during PMS. They are there because you need certain things that you aren't getting. Many people will say that the cause of PMS is something like low progesterone. That may be true in its own kind of reductionist way, but then there's the question of WHY is your progesterone low? It's because you haven't been listening to your body-mind. So you don't have to get diagnosed with something or know what's happening on the scientific level in order to know how to start feeling better.

So, how DO you start feeling better? There are basically three major areas you need to look at when trying to improve PMS. One is scheduling, one is food and herbs, and one is movement.

The first and potentially most important part for some people is the need to start slowing down, relaxing, and taking good care of yourself. If you don't, you are going to feel irritable and drained. Respect your body, respect what it needs, and it won't need to send you all these pain signals to get your attention so strongly. It's asking for you to slow down. The first thing you can do is to follow your cycle like I outlined in chapter three, especially during the luteal and menstrual phases.

The second issue is movement, so just go back to chapter five and make sure that you're following the suggestions. If you're not getting enough movement, you won't be detoxifying extra hormones efficiently, you'll have inflammation, and everything will be stagnant in you. That will contribute to cramps and mood swings and all the other crappy things that are making you and everyone around you miserable. At the same time, make sure you're not exercising too intensely, especially in your luteal and menstrual phases, because that will put too much stress on your body. It's common for elite female athletes to actually stop menstruating or get irregular cycles, because they're either pushing themselves down to too low of a body fat which results in very low levels of necessary hormones, or they're increasing their stress levels so much that their body is just shutting it down because reproduction isn't necessary or healthy when you're under stress. Your body interprets stress as getting chased by a tiger or some other immediate threat to life.

It's important to also be eating well so that your nutrient requirements are being met. Like I said in the food chapter, your body has higher requirements for many nutrients during the luteal and menstrual phases. I had also mentioned that women who have PMS eat about 275% more sugar than women who don't have PMS, so if you haven't already, kick the sugar habit.

There are also herbs that can help alleviate PMS. One of the most popular is chaste tree or chaste tree berry, also known as vitex. It helps fix menstrual irregularities and it also helps with PMS, because it raises the level of progesterone in the body. Progesterone is kind of like valium, it actually acts as a sedative and a feel-good or anti-anxiety hormone. You definitely don't want to be low on that.

Two other herbs that help with PMS are dong quai and maca. Maca is especially good for balancing hormones, and it's really easy to add to smoothies if you get the powder form. If you prefer capsules, you can also get it that way. Dong quai is supposed to not taste very good, so capsules might be best there.

One more herb that could be helpful for your overall menstrual health is raspberry leaf. It balances your hormones, relieves menstrual discomfort, and may increase your fertility. You can pick this yourself from wild raspberry plants, which are very common in most areas. The best time to pick them is in the late spring before they blossom. You can then dry and crush the leaves to have for tea. You can also simply buy raspberry leaf tea bags from health food stores or herb companies- some grocery stores even have it now.

If you have a lot of uncomfortable bloating, make sure you're watching what you eat, especially with sugar and dairy. Keep that food journal and try to make some connections between what you eat and how you feel. It may also help you to eat several small meals throughout the day instead of just a couple large ones. Dandelion and parsley act as natural diuretics, so eating them or making teas out of them could help.

I want to emphasize that while herbs are helpful companions to have, they're not the whole story. If you have PMS and are living off of doughnuts and soda and never take time to relax or be by yourself for your entire cycle, then taking an herb probably won't do much for you. Our bodies are holistic- everything affects everything else and you have to look at the whole picture.

Chapter 7:

Conclusion

The female menstrual cycle is a truly powerful gift. It reminds us that we are intricately connected to Gaia; we are, in fact, a part of her just as our cells are part of us. To me, this is a notion that's both humbling and empowering. Our bodies are sacred, expressing the infinite wisdom that can be represented through the ancient goddesses. Treat yourself as such- a goddess.

View yourself as a goddess with a sacred body. Get to know the intricacies of your monthly cycle. Listen to your body's messages and respect it by planning your activities in accordance with your strengths and energy levels. Feed yourself like a goddess. Move like a goddess. If you just shift your mindset like this, you can have a truly happy menstrual cycle. You'll be able to meet any challenges that come to you, you'll know that you're living with integrity, and you'll be a true example of feminine beauty and power.

There is an online course that accompanies this book. It gives you lifetime access to all the information in the book in audio and visual formats, plus downloads for a phase journal, a health tracker, and a fertility chart; a menstrual yoga video; access to a secret Facebook group exclusively for women in the course where you can talk to me and each other; and a monthly new moon goddess oracle card reading by me. If this sounds like it might be for you, please find out more information at BioFit.us.

About the Author

Briar Accalia is the creator of BioFit. She's an entrepreneur, a black belt in karate, an herbalist and a polymath who has a passion for self-improvement and living naturally. She enjoys reading, writing, dancing, photography, camping, and discussing philosophy and ecology. She currently lives in Virginia with her husband and daughter. You can find her at BioFit.us and on Facebook and Twitter @BriarAccalia